LIVER DISEASE DIET COOKBOOK

Delicious Recipes For Hepatitis, Cirrhosis, Detox Healing, And Optimal Health

DR ELIAN GRIFFIN

DISCLAIMER

The nutritional recommendations and recipes in this book are meant solely for informative reasons. They are not meant to replace the counsel, diagnosis, or care of a qualified medical expert. If you have any doubts about a medical condition or dietary requirements, you should always see your physician or another trained healthcare expert.

All reasonable efforts have been taken by the author and publisher to ensure that the information contained in this book is correct as of the date of publication. Recommendations may alter, though, as medical knowledge is always changing. When using any of the recipes or instructions found here, the user assumes all liability and assumes no risk, whether personal or otherwise. People who have certain dietary requirements or medical issues should speak with a healthcare provider for personalized guidance. The given recipes are only ideas; you may need to adjust them to suit your own nutritional needs, tastes, and tolerances.

When you use this book, you agree to release the publisher, the author, and their representatives from any liability for any claims, damages, liabilities, costs, or expenditures resulting from your use of the book.

TABLE OF CONTENTS

ABOUT THE BOOK

With its insightful introduction that explores the liver's vital functions, common liver diseases, and their symptoms, "Liver Disease Diet Cookbook" is a valuable resource for anyone managing liver disease. It emphasizes the importance of nutrition in maintaining liver health and outlines specific dietary goals tailored to support liver function and prevent further damage.

The book provides practical advice on incorporating recommended food groups, staying hydrated, and the potential role of supplements. It delves deeply into the nutritional requirements for liver health, emphasizing the essential nutrients needed for optimal liver function and foods to avoid.

Readers will also learn about food safety practices, necessary kitchen tools, and safe cooking techniques, ensuring that every meal prepared supports liver health. Finally, it offers helpful advice on batch cooking and meal prep, as well as ways to modify recipes for liver-friendly options.

Another important topic addressed in this cookbook is building a liver-friendly pantry, which includes strategies for stocking basic ingredients, interpreting food labels, and identifying alternatives for common ingredients. The book also offers advice on how to shop on a budget and arrange the pantry for easy access, making healthy eating both practical and economical.

Anyone managing liver disease needs to create balanced meal plans, and this book highlights the value of meal planning with sample plans and advice on variety and balance.

It also provides instructions on how to modify plans to accommodate various dietary requirements and monitor progress to make necessary modifications.

Along with hearty soup recipes, light salads, and tips for balanced salads, including homemade dressings and toppings, the cookbook offers a wide range of recipes that start with healthy breakfast options, quick and easy liver-friendly ideas, smoothies, whole grain choices, and protein-packed meals.

It also includes healthy snack options, liver-friendly dips and spreads, vegetable snacks, high-fiber choices, and smart snacking tips.

Special diet considerations are covered, offering advice for managing other health conditions, gluten-free recipes, dairy-free and vegan options, low-sodium recipes, and the ability to customize recipes to fit specific needs.

Beverages are another focus, with options for liver-friendly drinks, homemade juice and smoothie recipes, herbal teas, hydrating and detoxifying drinks, and advice on avoiding alcohol and sugary drinks.

The book emphasizes maintaining long-term dietary habits with strategies for building sustainable habits, tracking progress, staying motivated, dealing with setbacks, and continuing education and support. It also offers advice on how to prepare liver-friendly dishes for gatherings, navigate social situations, and communicate dietary needs effectively when dining out.

"Liver Disease Diet Cookbook" is a vital tool for anyone looking to manage liver disease through a deliberate and informed approach to nutrition, offering thorough guidance and support for a healthier lifestyle. Common concerns and FAQs address important questions like managing other health conditions, dealing with flare-ups, staying motivated, the role of supplements and handling dietary missteps.

CHAPTER ONE

AN OVERVIEW OF LIVER FUNCTIONS

The liver is an important organ that carries out numerous vital tasks that are necessary to preserve general health. Toxin removal from the bloodstream is one of its main functions; the liver breaks down and gets rid of harmful substances, making sure they are neutralized and removed from the body.

The liver also plays a vital role in metabolism, turning nutrients from food into energy and necessary biochemical substances. It also stores nutrients like glycogen, vitamins, and minerals, releasing them into the blood when needed to maintain energy levels and nutritional balance.

The liver also plays an important role in the breakdown of old or damaged red blood cells, the production of bile, which is required for the digestion and absorption of fats in the small intestine, the synthesis of blood clotting proteins, and the production of albumin, a protein that keeps fluid balance in the bloodstream. In addition, the liver regulates blood composition, making sure those levels of glucose, protein, and fat stay within healthy ranges, and it breaks down ammonia, a byproduct of protein metabolism, into urea, which is excreted by the kidneys.

Another amazing characteristic of the liver is its ability to regenerate. This means that the liver can heal itself and carry on with its vital functions even after it has been injured or become diseased. Knowing these functions emphasizes how important it is to maintain liver health with a healthy diet and way of life because the liver's proper function is essential to overall health and the body's ability to detoxify, metabolize, and maintain energy levels.

COMMON LIVER DISEASE TYPES

A wide range of conditions affect the liver's capacity to function normally. Hepatitis is one of the most prevalent types of liver disease.

Hepatitis is an inflammation of the liver brought on by viral infections (hepatitis A, B, C, D, and E), excessive alcohol consumption, or autoimmune responses. Chronic hepatitis can result in liver damage and scarring, which is referred to as cirrhosis.

Cirrhosis is frequently brought on by prolonged alcohol abuse, chronic hepatitis, or fatty liver disease. If left untreated, cirrhosis can eventually lead to liver failure.

Another common liver condition is non-alcoholic fatty liver disease (NAFLD), which is more common in people who have metabolic syndrome, obesity, or diabetes.

NAFLD is characterized by the buildup of excess fat in the liver cells, which can lead to non-alcoholic steatohepatitis (NASH), which causes inflammation and damage to the liver cells; if NASH is not treated, it can result in cirrhosis and liver cancer. Since cirrhosis and chronic liver disease are frequently the precursors of liver cancer, early detection and management of liver conditions are essential for preventing the development of cancer.

Understanding these common liver diseases emphasizes the need for awareness, early diagnosis, and effective management to maintain liver health and prevent life-threatening complications.

Other notable liver diseases include autoimmune liver diseases like primary biliary cholangitis (PBC) and autoimmune hepatitis, where the body's immune system mistakenly attacks liver cells; these conditions require careful monitoring and treatment to prevent progression to more severe liver damage and complications.

SIGNS AND PROGNOSIS

Liver disease symptoms can vary greatly depending on the particular condition and how severe it is, but there are some common indicators that something may be wrong with the liver. One of the most common symptoms of liver disease is jaundice, which is a yellowing of the skin and eyes.

This is caused by the buildup of bilirubin, a byproduct of red blood cell breakdown. Other symptoms include fatigue, weakness, and unexplained weight loss. Abdominal pain or swelling, especially in the upper right side of the body where the liver is located, as well as pale stool, dark urine, and itching.

The process of diagnosing liver disease usually consists of a review of the patient's medical history, a physical examination, blood tests (liver function tests, for example), and imaging studies (ultrasound, CT scan, MRI, etc.).

Blood tests, like liver function tests, measure levels of liver enzymes, bilirubin, and proteins to assess liver health and identify abnormalities; elevated liver enzymes can indicate inflammation or damage). Imaging studies (liver biopsy, etc.) provide detailed visuals of the liver's structure and can be used to diagnose specific liver conditions and determine the extent of liver damage.

Effective management and treatment of liver disease depend on early diagnosis and detection. People who are at higher risk of liver disease because of obesity, excessive alcohol consumption, or a family history of the disease should have their liver health regularly monitored to identify problems early.

By quickly seeking medical attention when symptoms appear, people can take proactive measures to manage their liver disease, minimize complications, and preserve their general health.

DIET IS IMPORTANT FOR LIVER HEALTH

Diet is a critical component of liver health and liver disease management. A balanced diet gives the liver the necessary nutrients to carry out its many functions. Dietary changes can lessen the burden on the liver, encourage healing, and stop further damage in liver disease patients.

Avoiding processed foods, unhealthy fats, and sugars, which can aggravate fatty liver disease and inflammation, and instead focusing on whole foods, fruits, vegetables, whole grains, lean proteins, and healthy fats, can help support liver health.

Some specific nutrients and foods are particularly good for liver function: foods high in antioxidants, like berries, nuts, and leafy greens, help shield liver cells from damage caused by free radicals; foods high in omega-3 fatty acids, like salmon and flaxseeds, have anti-inflammatory qualities that can help people with liver conditions; foods high in fiber help with digestion and blood sugar regulation, which lowers the risk of developing non-alcoholic fatty liver disease; and drinking enough water is crucial for liver detoxification and general liver health.

Tailored dietary approaches are often required for individuals with particular liver diseases. For example, people with cirrhosis may need to restrict their sodium intake to avoid fluid retention and swelling, while people with hepatitis may benefit from increasing their protein intake to support tissue repair.

Speaking with a healthcare professional or registered dietitian can assist in developing a customized diet plan that takes into account each individual's specific needs and ensures that dietary choices support liver health and contribute to overall well-being.

THE LIVER DISEASE DIET'S OBJECTIVES

Maintaining a steady supply of nutrients through a balanced diet helps people maintain stable blood sugar levels, prevent malnutrition, and support the liver's regenerative processes.

The main goals of a liver disease diet are to support liver function and promote healing while preventing further damage. One important goal is to reduce the workload of the liver by providing easily digestible nutrients that do not strain the liver's metabolic capacity. This involves consuming smaller, more frequent meals and avoiding heavy, high-fat foods that can overburden the liver.

Avoiding alcohol, which can worsen liver damage, is also crucial for people with liver disease. Certain dietary restrictions, like cutting back on sodium intake for those with cirrhosis, help manage symptoms and prevent complications like fluid retention and swelling. Monitoring and adjusting nutrient intake based on individual needs and the progression of liver disease are vital aspects of managing liver health through diet. Reducing inflammation and promoting liver cell repair is another important goal that can be accomplished by including anti-inflammatory foods, such as fruits, vegetables, whole grains, and healthy fats, into the diet.

Finally, a diet for liver disease should promote overall health and well-being by strengthening the body's defenses against infections and other health problems that could result from liver dysfunction.

This comprehensive strategy includes keeping a healthy weight, exercising frequently, and implementing lifestyle changes that improve general health. By concentrating on these objectives, people with liver disease can enhance their quality of life, better manage their symptoms, and possibly even slow down the progression of liver damage, which could lead to better long-term outcomes.

CHAPTER TWO

THE NEEDS OF NUTRITION FOR LIVER HEALTH

CRUCIAL ELEMENTS FOR HEALTHY LIVER FUNCTION

A diet rich in leafy greens, dairy products, nuts, and fish is essential for maintaining the health of the liver, which is an organ responsible for many functions like detoxification, protein synthesis, and the production of biochemicals needed for digestion. The liver also needs a variety of essential nutrients, and vitamins like A, D, E, and K are critical for liver health. Vitamin A supports the immune system and tissue repair, while vitamin D is essential for calcium absorption and bone health. Vitamin E acts as an antioxidant, protecting liver cells from damage. Finally, vitamin K is necessary for blood clotting and bone metabolism.

Eat foods high in seafood, meat, nuts, and seeds to help maintain the health and functionality of your liver. Minerals like zinc and selenium have important roles in liver function. Zinc is involved in over 300 enzyme reactions, including those crucial for liver metabolism and immune function. Selenium, another potent antioxidant, helps prevent cellular damage by neutralizing free radicals.

Lean meats, eggs, dairy, legumes, and nuts are high-quality protein sources that provide the amino acids needed for liver repair and regeneration. A diet high in these nutrients will support the liver's ability to carry out its many functions efficiently. Proteins are another essential nutrient for the liver because they help repair liver cells and produce hormones and enzymes.

ITEMS TO STEER CLEAR OF

Foods like fried foods, fast food, and high-fat dairy products should be avoided to maintain optimal liver health. Healthy fats, like those found in avocados, nuts, and olive oil, can support liver function without harming it. High-fat foods, especially those high in saturated and trans fats, can lead to fat accumulation in the liver and potentially cause fatty liver disease.

Additional culprits that can harm liver health include sugar and refined carbohydrates; excessive sugar intake can cause insulin resistance and liver fat accumulation. Refined sugar-containing foods like candies, pastries, sodas, and white bread should be avoided in favor of whole grains, fruits, and vegetables, which offer essential nutrients without the negative effects of refined sugars.

One of the most well-known substances to stay away from for liver health is alcohol. Drinking too much alcohol can cause fatty liver disease, cirrhosis, and inflammation of the liver. To protect the liver, limit or stay away from alcohol completely. If you do drink, moderation is key; try to stick to recommendations that limit it to one drink for women and two for men per day.

SUGGESTED FOOD GROUPS

Incorporating a range of food groups that offer balanced nutrition is crucial for supporting liver health. Fruits and vegetables are a great source of antioxidants, vitamins, and minerals that help with liver detoxification and repair. Leafy greens, berries, and citrus fruits are especially helpful as they reduce inflammation and shield liver cells from harm.

Oats, brown rice, and quinoa are examples of whole grains that are great for liver health because they contain fiber, which helps with digestion and keeps you at a healthy weight, which lessens the strain on your liver. Whole grains also help control blood sugar levels, which lowers your chance of developing fatty liver disease.

Lean proteins—found in chicken, turkey, fish, beans, and legumes—are essential for liver function because they supply the amino acids needed for liver repair and enzyme synthesis. Fish—particularly omega-3 fatty acids-rich varieties like salmon and sardines—helps lower inflammation and liver fat accumulation. Including these food groups in daily meals can help guarantee that the liver gets the nourishment it needs to function at its best.

Maintaining adequate hydration supports the kidneys, which work in tandem with the liver to remove toxins from the bloodstream. Aim for a minimum of eight glasses of water per day, or more if you are physically active or live in a hot climate. Water is essential for the liver's detoxification processes, aiding in the removal of waste products and toxins from the body.

Teas made from milk thistle, dandelion root, and green tea have been shown to have liver-protective properties. These herbal teas can help reduce inflammation, promote liver cell regeneration, and enhance the liver's detoxification processes. Including a variety of these teas in your daily routine can provide benefits beyond hydration. Herbal teas and infusions can also support liver health while keeping you hydrated.

Water is the best beverage to stay hydrated, but you should also avoid sugar-filled drinks and alcohol as much as possible, as these can aggravate liver damage and cause other health problems.

To stay properly hydrated and support liver function, stick to drinking water and herbal teas or other low-calorie beverages.

FUNCTION OF ADD-ONS

The most well-known supplement for liver health is milk thistle, which comes in capsule and tea form. It contains silymarin, an antioxidant and anti-inflammatory compound that can help protect liver cells from damage and promote regeneration. Supplements can play a supportive role in maintaining liver health, especially when dietary intake of certain nutrients is inadequate.

Zinc and selenium supplements can support liver metabolism and protect against oxidative stress; B vitamins, including B12 and folate, are essential for liver detoxification and overall function; and vitamin and mineral supplements can be helpful, especially if there are dietary deficiencies. However, it is important to see a doctor before beginning any supplementation to ensure proper dosage and prevent potential drug interactions.

For people with non-alcoholic fatty liver disease (NAFLD), omega-3 fatty acids, which are commonly taken as fish oil supplements, can help lower inflammation and fat accumulation in the liver. However, as with any supplement, it is important to follow dosage recommendations and speak with a healthcare provider to ensure safety and effectiveness.

CHAPTER THREE

SAFE COOKING TECHNIQUES

For those on a diet for liver disease, safe cooking techniques are essential because they preserve the integrity of nutrients and minimize the formation of potentially harmful substances. Steaming is one of the best techniques because it retains vitamins and minerals and doesn't add fat. To steam vegetables or fish, use a steamer basket, place the food above boiling water, cover, and cook until it's tender. Poaching is another great technique, especially for proteins like chicken or fish. Cook the protein gently until it's done, simmering the water or broth to minimize fat and prevent the formation of potentially harmful compounds that occur when cooking at high temperatures.

Baking is another safe method that works well with vegetables, lean meats, and fish because it retains moisture and nutrients even when cooked at lower temperatures. Sautéing with little to no oil is another safe method that works well with vegetables, meats, and fish because it's quick and helps lock in flavor without using too much fat or calories. Non-stick pans or a light coating of heart-healthy oils like olive or avocado oil are good options.

Finally, grilling can be beneficial to liver health if done properly. Meals prepared with these techniques will be safe and nutritious, supporting liver health. Avoid charring meats, as this creates hazardous chemicals. Instead, use moderate heat and keep the grill clean to prevent flare-ups. You can also control exposure to direct flames by wrapping foods in foil or using a grill basket.

ESSENTIAL UTENSILS FOR THE KITCHEN

To follow a liver disease diet, you must have the right equipment in your kitchen. A good set of non-stick cookware minimizes the need for extra fats to be added during cooking, which encourages healthier meal preparation.

Look for non-stick pans, baking sheets, and muffin tins. A food processor or blender helps make smoothies, purees, and soups, which makes it easier for you to include more fruits and vegetables in your diet.

Efficient preparation of fresh ingredients requires sharp knives and a sturdy cutting board; measuring cups and spoons guarantee accurate portion control, which is critical for controlling nutrient intake; silicone spatulas and tongs facilitate stirring and flipping food without marring non-stick surfaces; and for those who like batch cooking, purchase airtight containers in different sizes to store prepared meals and leftovers, which will help you stay on track with your diet.

Last but not least, for easy, hands-off cooking, think about an instant pot or slow cooker. These appliances are great for making wholesome, one-pot meals that can cook slowly over time, retaining flavor and nutrients. They are especially helpful for people who are busy and want to maintain a diet that is liver-healthy without spending hours in the kitchen.

With the right tools, cooking meals that are liver-healthy becomes easier and more pleasurable.

Food safety and hygiene must be upheld at all times, but especially during a liver disease diet. Always wash your hands well with soap and water before handling any food. Sanitize and clean all kitchen surfaces, such as countertops, cutting boards, and utensils, to prevent cross-contamination. Use different cutting boards for raw meats and vegetables to prevent the spread of harmful bacteria. Keep your kitchen clean and hygienic by routinely cleaning and disinfecting kitchen towels and sponges.

To prevent foodborne illnesses and spoilage, it is important to store food properly. Perishable items, like meats, dairy products, and cut fruits and vegetables, should be refrigerated within two hours of purchase or preparation. It is also important to keep your refrigerator at the proper temperature, which is usually below 40°F (4°C).

Label leftovers with dates so you can keep track of their freshness and consume them within safe time frames. Freezing is a great way to extend the shelf life of prepared meals and ingredients.

Follow strict food safety and hygiene guidelines to protect your health and effectively support your liver-friendly diet. Cooking foods to their safe internal temperatures is crucial to killing any harmful bacteria. Use a food thermometer to ensure meats are cooked through. For example, poultry should reach an internal temperature of 165°F (74°C). Steer clear of raw or undercooked foods, particularly eggs, meats, and seafood.

TIPS FOR BATCH COOKING AND MEAL PREP

The following tips will help make a liver disease diet easier to follow and more time-efficient: plan your meals for the week, choosing recipes that follow liver health guidelines; make a shopping list based on these recipes to make sure you have all the ingredients on hand; set aside a specific time, like Sunday afternoon, to cook multiple meals at once; this will help you stick to your diet and lessen the daily burden of meal preparation.

To keep precooked meals fresh, buy high-quality storage containers. Glass containers with airtight lids work best because they don't leak and can be used to reheat food in the microwave. Label each container with the contents and the date so you know what has to be eaten first.

You can also divide meals into single-serving portions so that it's convenient to grab a nutritious meal or snack on the go. Soups, stews, and casseroles are great to batch cook because they freeze and reheat well.

Preparing meals ahead of time ensures that healthy, liver-friendly options are always available, making it easier to maintain a balanced diet. Variety is key to preventing meal fatigue, so incorporate different proteins, vegetables, and grains in your batch cooking. Try making a large batch of brown rice or quinoa and using it as a base for various dishes throughout the week. Roasted vegetables, grilled chicken, and bean salads are versatile options that can be mixed and matched.

MODIFYING DISHES TO PROMOTE LIVER HEALTH

Making thoughtful substitutions to lower fat, sugar, and sodium while increasing nutritional value is part of modifying recipes for liver health. Some healthy substitutions include switching from high-fat to low-fat dairy products, replacing butter with olive or avocado oil when cooking, and choosing lean proteins like chicken, fish, and plant-based options like beans and lentils instead of red or processed meats.

Cutting back on sodium consumption is essential for liver health. Instead of adding salt to your food, flavor it with herbs, spices, and citrus juices. Dried or fresh herbs like thyme, basil, and oregano add strong flavors without raising blood pressure. Try different spices like cumin, paprika, and turmeric to add complexity and depth to your dishes.

If you use canned beans or vegetables, make sure they are low-sodium varieties or rinse them well to get rid of excess salt.

Add more fruits and vegetables to your recipes to increase fiber, vitamins, and antioxidants that support liver function. Replace refined grains with whole grains, such as brown rice, quinoa, and whole-wheat pasta; these grains offer more nutrients and fiber that support overall health and digestion. With these small changes, you can turn classic recipes into nutrient-dense, delicious, and liver-friendly versions.

CHAPTER FOUR

CONSTRUCTING A LIVER-FRIENDLY CLOSET

KEEPING KEY INGREDIENTS IN STOCK

Building a liver-friendly pantry begins with stockpiling basic ingredients that promote liver health. Whole grains, such as quinoa, brown rice, and oats, are staples because they are high in fiber and nutrients that support liver function and digestion. Add a variety of legumes, like chickpeas, lentils, and black beans, as they are excellent sources of plant-based protein and provide essential minerals like iron and magnesium. Fresh and frozen veggies, especially leafy greens, broccoli, and beets, are essential because they are packed with compounds and antioxidants that support liver detoxification.

Lean proteins, such as chicken, turkey, and fish like salmon and mackerel, provide essential amino acids and omega-3 fatty acids that help repair and regenerate liver cells.

Fresh fruits, especially berries, apples, and citrus fruits, should also be on hand as they are rich in vitamins and antioxidants. Healthy fats, such as those found in olive oil, avocado oil, and nuts like almonds and walnuts, help reduce inflammation and support overall liver function.

With their anti-inflammatory and detoxifying qualities, herbs and spices like parsley, turmeric, garlic, and ginger belong in your pantry. You can flavor your food without adding too much salt by using low-sodium broths and stocks. By stocking your pantry with these ingredients, you can be sure that you'll always have the ingredients for healthy, liver-friendly meals on hand.

EXAMINING AND INTERPRETING NUTRITION LABELS

Maintaining a liver-friendly diet requires reading and comprehending food labels. Start by paying attention to the ingredient list; search for whole, minimally processed ingredients and steer clear of products with a lengthy list of additives and preservatives. The ingredients are listed in order of weight, meaning that the first few items are the most prevalent in the product. Items that contain hydrogenated oils, high-fructose corn syrup, and artificial colors should be avoided as they may be detrimental to liver health.

The nutritional information panel should then be examined. It is crucial to limit sugar, sodium, and saturated fats in a diet that is liver-friendly. Products with healthier fats and low levels of added sugars should be sought after. Additionally, a higher fiber content can aid in better digestion and overall liver function, so products with at least 3-5 grams of fiber per serving should be prioritized.

Mastering food labels will help you make decisions that support liver health. Another important skill is understanding serving sizes. A lot of packaged foods list nutritional information based on a serving size that is much smaller than what you might eat. Be sure to multiply the nutritional values by the number of servings you are likely to consume to get an accurate picture of your intake.

Changing common ingredients to liver-friendly ones can make a big difference in your diet. For example, whole grain or almond flour, which are higher in fiber and nutrients and support better liver function, can be used in place of refined white flour in baking and cooking. Natural sweeteners like honey, maple syrup, or stevia can also be used in place of white sugar because they are less harsh on the liver and have more health benefits.

If you love to cook with cream, coconut cream is a great substitute that adds richness without the unhealthy fats found in dairy cream. For dairy products, think about using plant-based alternatives like almond milk, coconut milk, or oat milk. These options are often lower in fat and easier for the liver to process. Opt for avocado or olive oil instead of butter, which provides healthy fats that can help reduce liver inflammation.

In terms of protein, you can enjoy your favorite recipes while adhering to a diet that supports liver function and overall wellness by substituting lean poultry, fish, or plant-based proteins like tofu and tempeh. These options are lower in saturated fats and contain beneficial nutrients that support liver health.

SOME ADVICE FOR FRUGAL SHOPPING

Eating healthily doesn't have to break the bank. To start, figure out what you need for each meal and create a shopping list based on those ingredients. This will help you stay away from impulsive purchases and make sure you buy only what you need. Whenever possible, buy in bulk, especially for staples like whole grains, legumes, nuts, and seeds, which are often less expensive when bought in larger quantities and preserved well.

Buying seasonal produce can help you save money and get fresher, healthier produce. You can find seasonal fruits and vegetables at lower costs at local farmers' markets. You can also buy frozen produce, which is often less expensive than fresh and can be stored for a longer period, saving you waste and guaranteeing you always have healthy options on hand.

Generic or store-brand products are often less expensive than name-brand products and are of similar quality; finally, try to minimize the purchase of pre-packaged and processed foods, which can be more expensive and less healthy. By using coupons and keeping an eye out for sales and discounts, you can keep a liver-friendly pantry without going over budget.

PUTTING YOUR PANTRY FOR EASY ACCESS

To prepare liver-friendly meals, it can be easier to organize your pantry. Start by putting similar items in groups, such as grains, legumes, nuts, and spices. For dry goods, such as rice, oats, and beans, use clear containers, which will keep them fresh longer and make it easier to see what you have at a glance. Label these containers with the contents and expiration dates to prevent confusion and waste.

Store less frequently used items on higher or lower shelves; this arrangement guarantees that you can find what you need quickly without having to search through the entire pantry.

Use baskets or bins to organize smaller items like spice packets, snacks, or tea bags. This keeps the pantry neat and prevents items from getting lost or buried. Arrange your pantry so that the most frequently used items are at eye level and easy to reach.

Maintaining an organized pantry can help you expedite your cooking process and guarantee that you always have the ingredients needed for liver-friendly meals. You can also consider using a rotating system where newer items are placed behind older ones. This first-in, first-out approach helps ensure that ingredients are used before they expire. Keep a running inventory of your pantry staples and check for items that need to be replenished regularly.

CHAPTER FIVE

MEAL PLANNING AND PREPARATION

THE VALUE OF MEAL PREPARATION

When it comes to managing liver disease, having a well-organized meal plan is essential. Planning meals ahead of time and carefully choosing your ingredients will help you maintain a balanced diet that supports liver health, lowers the risk of complications, and helps manage symptoms. It also helps prevent nutrient deficiencies that can arise from dietary restrictions and guarantees that meals are both enjoyable and nutritious.

Planning meals enables you to steer clear of high-fat, high-sugar, and high-sodium foods that can be harmful to liver health and instead concentrate on including more fruits, vegetables, lean proteins, and whole grains, which are beneficial for liver function and overall well-being. Eating a variety of food groups in appropriate portions is often necessary when it comes to providing essential nutrients like proteins, carbohydrates, fats, vitamins, and minerals, which are crucial for overall health and liver function.

Meal planning ensures that you are consuming the appropriate amount of calories and nutrients for your particular health condition, which makes it easier to stick to a liver-friendly diet and promote long-term liver health.

Additionally, meal planning helps with portion sizes and prevents overeating, which is essential for maintaining a healthy weight. Overweight and obesity can lead to non-alcoholic fatty liver disease (NAFLD) and other liver-related issues.

ADVICE ON KEEPING THINGS BALANCED AND DIVERSE

You can make sure you get all the nutrients you need by including a variety of fruits and vegetables in your meal plans. Try to include as many different colors and types of vegetables as you can. This will add interest to your meals and guarantee that you get a wide range of vitamins, minerals, and antioxidants that support liver health. You can also get a broad spectrum of nutrients by combining different types of vegetables, like leafy greens, cruciferous vegetables, and root vegetables.

Another key component of meal planning is including a variety of protein sources. Lean proteins, like turkey, chicken, fish, tofu, legumes, and eggs, can be switched up to offer diversity and essential amino acids. Fish, particularly fatty fish like salmon and mackerel, is especially helpful because it contains omega-3 fatty acids, which have anti-inflammatory qualities and can support liver health. Plant-based proteins, like beans, lentils, and quinoa, can also be included to provide diversity and fiber, which is essential for both liver health and digestion.

Whole grains, like brown rice, quinoa, oats, and whole wheat bread, provide vital nutrients and fiber that help regulate blood sugar levels and support digestive health. Healthy fats, like those found in avocados, nuts, seeds, and olive oil, can support liver health without overburdening it.

By combining these different food groups and rotating them throughout the week, you can create meal plans that are nutritious, enjoyable, and balanced.

Customized meal plans that meet specific dietary requirements can be made possible by taking into account the individual's needs and preferences, as well as their condition, nutritional needs, and food tolerances.

For example, a person with cirrhosis may need to limit their protein intake to prevent hepatic encephalopathy, while a person with fatty liver disease may benefit from a higher protein diet to support weight loss and muscle maintenance.

When creating meal plans, it's important to take into account any co-existing medical conditions, such as diabetes or hypertension. For instance, if you have both diabetes and liver disease, you should control your carbohydrate intake and prioritize foods low in the

Glycemic index to keep your blood sugar stable. In these situations, adding more non-starchy vegetables, whole grains, and lean proteins can help create balanced meals that address both conditions at the same time. Similarly, if you have hypertension, you should cut back on sodium and emphasize foods high in potassium, like bananas, sweet potatoes, and spinach.

Furthermore, meal plans should be sufficiently flexible to account for changes in preferences and lifestyle. This could involve organizing meals that are simple to make on busy days or incorporating favorite dishes in a liver-friendly way.

For example, if you're a pasta lover, choosing whole grain or legume-based pasta with a low-fat sauce that's rich in vegetables can make pasta fit for a liver-friendly diet. Meal plans that are flexible and personalized can be more enjoyable and sustainable, which improves adherence and results in better health outcomes.

Maintaining a successful meal plan for liver disease requires tracking your progress. Recording your meals and any symptoms you encounter can help you understand how different foods affect your liver condition, enabling you to make more informed choices. You can monitor what you eat, how much, and how often by keeping a food diary or using a meal planning app. This practice allows you to identify patterns, make necessary adjustments, and ensure you are sticking to your nutritional goals.

Consultation with a healthcare provider or dietitian regularly can provide valuable insights and help fine-tune your meal plan based on your ongoing health status and nutritional needs. For example, you can modify your plan to exclude certain foods that cause discomfort or adverse symptoms and find suitable alternatives. Regularly reviewing your meal plan and making adjustments based on your progress is essential.

This may involve increasing or decreasing certain nutrients, changing portion sizes, or introducing new foods to keep your diet balanced and interesting.

Adjustments also include adjusting to changes in your lifestyle or health condition. Your dietary needs may change as your liver health improves or if you face new health challenges. Being proactive and adaptable in your meal planning approach guarantees that you can effectively adjust to these changes. For instance, you may need to modify your calorie intake to maintain your new weight if you reach your weight loss goals. Ongoing monitoring and modification of your meal plan helps sustain its efficacy and support long-term liver health.

THE VALUE OF A BALANCED BREAKFAST

A balanced breakfast jump-starts the metabolism and replenishes the body with vital nutrients after an overnight fast; for those with liver conditions, it is critical to eat foods that support liver function and aid in liver recovery; for those managing liver disease, a nutritious breakfast is essential for maintaining overall health, particularly for those who are managing blood sugar spikes that can stress the liver and other organs.

Foods high in antioxidants, fiber, and healthy fats can reduce inflammation and support the liver's ability to repair itself. Eating a nutrient-dense breakfast helps ensure that the body receives adequate vitamins and minerals, which are essential for the liver's detoxification processes. Including a variety of food groups in breakfast can help meet daily nutritional needs and improve overall health outcomes for those with liver disease.

A nutritious and enjoyable breakfast can also help set a positive tone for the rest of the day, encouraging healthier eating habits overall. Furthermore, a regular and healthy breakfast routine can improve medication efficacy for patients with liver disease by promoting better absorption of nutrients and medications.

This routine helps establish a balanced diet that contributes to maintaining a healthy weight, which is critical in managing liver disease.

SIMPLE AND FAST BREAKFAST IDEAS THAT ARE LIVER-FRIENDLY

Meal planning for people with liver disease can be made easier by coming up with quick and healthy breakfast options. Avocado toast, for example, is made with half an avocado mashed on whole-grain toast and topped with a sprinkle of flaxseeds. Flaxseeds add fiber and omega-3 fatty acids, which help reduce inflammation, and avocados are rich in antioxidants and healthy fats that support liver health.

An additional simple recipe is a vegetable omelet. Eggs are an excellent source of high-quality protein and choline, both of which are good for liver function. Beat a few eggs with a little milk, then pour into a hot pan and add chopped veggies such as bell peppers, tomatoes, and spinach. Cook until set, fold in half, and serve. This breakfast is ready in less than ten minutes and offers a good combination of vitamins and protein.

If you'd rather have something sweet for breakfast, try making overnight oats. Just put rolled oats, chia seeds, and a dash of cinnamon in a jar and refrigerate overnight. The next morning, top with fresh berries and a drizzle of honey. This is a high-fiber, antioxidant-rich meal that supports liver detoxification and general health. Since it can be made ahead of time, overnight oats are a convenient and liver-friendly option for hectic mornings.

SHAKES & SMOOTHIES FOR HEPATIC HEALTH

Smoothies and shakes are great breakfast options for liver health because they offer a concentrated dose of nutrients in a convenient, easily digested form. A green smoothie that contains banana, spinach, kale, and a splash of coconut water can be especially helpful because the antioxidants and chlorophyll in the spinach and kale help cleanse the liver, and the potassium in the bananas supports liver function.

Try a berry smoothie with Greek yogurt for a high-protein option. Blend a cup of mixed berries, a scoop of Greek yogurt, and a splash of almond milk. Greek yogurt adds protein and probiotics to help with digestion and nutrient absorption, and berries are high in antioxidants and vitamins that support liver health. This smoothie is delicious and nutritious, making it a great way to start the day.

The anti-inflammatory qualities of turmeric and ginger, along with the natural sweetness and potassium provided by the frozen banana, can all be found in a liver-friendly shake. In a blender, combine a cup of unsweetened almond milk, a tablespoon of almond butter, a teaspoon of turmeric, a small piece of ginger, and a frozen banana. This shake offers a well-balanced combination of nutrients that support liver health and overall wellness.

WHOLE GRAIN SELECTIONS

A diet rich in whole grains is essential for liver health, as they provide fiber and nutrients that support liver function and overall health. A bowl of steel-cut oatmeal in the morning can boost digestion and provide sustained energy. Oats are high in beta-glucan, a soluble fiber type that lowers cholesterol and improves liver health. Garnish with nuts and fresh fruit for extra nutrition and flavor.

Another great whole-grain option for breakfast is quinoa. Because it is high in fiber and contains all nine essential amino acids, it is a complete protein that is great for liver health. To make a savory dish that is both filling and nutritious, try making a quinoa breakfast bowl with sautéed vegetables, a poached egg, and a drizzle of olive oil.

Additionally, whole-grain bread can be included in liver-friendly breakfasts. For example, try whole-grain toast with sliced bananas and a spread of almond butter. The complex carbohydrates and fiber in whole grain bread help to stabilize blood sugar levels, and the protein and healthy fats in almond butter add to the meal, which is quick and filling and promotes liver health as well as general well-being.

HIGH-PROTEIN BREAKFASTS

For those who are managing liver disease, eating a high-protein breakfast is essential because it aids in tissue repair and supports liver function. One high-protein option is a tofu scramble. Crumble firm tofu into a pan with a small amount of olive oil, add turmeric and cumin, and cook until the tofu is heated through and the vegetables are tender. This plant-based breakfast offers a significant amount of antioxidants and protein to support liver health.

A protein-rich breakfast option is a salad of diced avocado, cherry tomatoes, red onion, and arugula mixed with smoked salmon slices. Drizzle with olive oil and lemon juice to create a light, nutrient-rich dish. The fatty acids in the avocado add fiber and healthy fats, while the smoked salmon provides high-quality protein and omega-3 fatty acids that support liver function and reduce inflammation.

For a quick and easy way to up your protein intake, try a cottage cheese bowl with fresh berries, almonds, and honey on top of a serving of low-fat cottage cheese. Cottage cheese is high in casein protein, which breaks down slowly and releases amino acids steadily, which is good for liver maintenance and repair. The berries and almonds also provide antioxidants and healthy fats, so this breakfast is satisfying and nutritious.

OPTIONS FOR HEALTHFUL SNACKS

Making nutritious snacks is crucial to managing liver disease because every bite should be easy on the liver. Try to stick to natural sugars and fiber from fresh fruit slices (apples, pears, and berries are great options because they are full of vitamins and antioxidants). Yogurt with a handful of nuts or seeds is also a great option because it provides gut health probiotics and healthy fats that support liver function. If you want to avoid added sugars, go for plain, unsweetened yogurt.

The key is to balance the fruits and vegetables so that each serving provides a variety of nutrients. Smoothies are another adaptable and liver-friendly snack. Blend ingredients like spinach, kale, bananas, and a small amount of avocado for a creamy texture. Add some chia seeds or flaxseeds for an extra boost of omega-3 fatty acids, which are beneficial for reducing inflammation. Use unsweetened almond milk or water as the base to keep it light and hydrating.

When made with whole oats, dried fruits, and a small amount of honey or maple syrup, homemade granola bars can also be a liver-friendly snack. You can add nuts and seeds for crunch and protein. You can control the ingredients by making your granola bars at home, avoiding the excessive sugars and additives that are often found in store-bought versions. These snacks are easy to pack for a quick, healthy option on the go.

SPREADS AND DIPS SAFE FOR LIVER

Made from chickpeas, tahini, lemon juice, and garlic, hummus is a fantastic option that is rich in fiber and plant-based protein, supporting digestive health and providing steady energy. Making hummus at home allows you to control the salt and avoid preservatives, keeping it as healthy as possible. Dips and spreads can be delicious and liver-friendly, ideal for pairing with fresh vegetables or whole-grain crackers.

Another great dip for liver disease sufferers is guacamole, which is made with avocados, lime juice, tomatoes, onions, and cilantro.

Rich in antioxidants and healthy fats, avocados' monounsaturated fats help lower inflammation in the liver and support overall liver health. Guacamole goes well with raw vegetable sticks, such as cucumber, carrot, and bell pepper sticks, for a wholesome, liver-friendly snack.

Greek yogurt is high in protein and lower in sugar than regular yogurt, making it a great choice for those managing liver disease. Yogurt-based dips, like tzatziki, are also beneficial. Made from Greek yogurt, cucumber, garlic, and dill, tzatziki is light, refreshing, and full of probiotics that aid in gut health. These dips taste great and also provide essential nutrients that support liver function.

CRUNCHY, FRESH VEGETABLE SNACKS

Including fresh, crunchy vegetables in your snack diet is an easy yet powerful way to support liver health. Low in calories but high in vitamins, minerals, and fiber, vegetables like carrots, celery, bell peppers, and cucumbers support the liver's detoxification processes and reduce inflammation. These vegetables are also easy to grab and snack on throughout the day when sliced into sticks or rounds.

You can add healthy fats and antioxidants to vegetables and make them taste better by pairing them with dips that are good for your liver, like guacamole or hummus. As an example, carrot sticks dipped in hummus have a satisfying crunch and provide a boost of fiber and protein, while bell pepper slices with guacamole offer a refreshing combination of healthy fats and antioxidants.

Making your veggie chips is another way to enjoy veggies: thinly slice veggies like sweet potatoes, beets, or zucchini, toss them lightly in olive oil and a little sea salt, and bake until crispy for a delicious and healthy alternative to store-bought chips. Because homemade veggie chips are lower in fat and additives that are bad for your liver, they're a great snack to keep your liver healthy.

A simple and delicious high-fiber snack is a serving of mixed nuts and seeds. Almonds, walnuts, chia seeds, and flaxseeds are great options, as they provide a mix of fiber, healthy fats, and protein. These nutrients help reduce inflammation and support overall liver function. Be mindful of portion sizes, as nuts and seeds are high in calories. High-fiber snacks are essential for maintaining liver health because they help regulate blood sugar levels and support digestive health.

In addition to being high in fiber, whole fruits like apples, pears, and strawberries also make convenient snacks. Pears and apples in particular are rich in pectin, a soluble fiber type that facilitates digestion and helps the liver process toxins.

Strawberries, blueberries, and raspberries are full of fiber and antioxidants that support liver health and lower oxidative stress. You can eat these fruits raw or blend them into yogurt or smoothies for a healthy snack.

Homemade oatmeal cookies are another fantastic high-fiber snack option. All you need are rolled oats, a tiny bit of honey or maple syrup, and add-ins like raisins, nuts, and a dash of cinnamon.

These cookies offer a substantial amount of fiber, which is good for liver health and digestion, and they provide a satisfying treat without the excess sugar and bad fats found in store-bought versions. Make a batch at home to have a convenient, healthy snack on hand.

TIPS FOR SMART SNACKING

Managing liver disease and making sure your body gets the nutrients it needs depends on how you snack. One important strategy is to prepare your snacks in advance. Having snacks ready, such as chopped vegetables, portioned nuts, and homemade dips, makes it easier to choose healthy options when hunger strikes.

This preparation also helps you avoid reaching for processed, unhealthy snacks that can damage your liver.

Another key component of smart snacking is portion control. Though even healthy snacks can cause weight gain if overindulged in, portioning out nuts, fruits, and vegetables using small containers or snack-sized bags helps control calorie intake and prevent overeating, which is important for maintaining a healthy weight and supporting liver function. Mindful portioning guarantees you're getting the right amount of nutrients without excess calories.

By following these wise snacking tips, you can enjoy healthy snacks that support liver wellness and overall health. Finally, pay attention to your body's hunger cues and avoid snacking out of boredom or habit. Eating only when you're genuinely hungry helps prevent unnecessary calorie consumption and supports overall health. Select snacks that provide a balance of protein, fiber, and healthy fats to keep you satisfied and energized. Combining these macronutrients helps stabilize blood sugar levels and supports liver health.

SALADS AND SOUPS ARE BENEFICIAL FOR LIVER HEALTH

Because they are nutrient-dense and hydrating, soups and salads are great options for supporting liver health. Soups, especially those made with a variety of vegetables and lean proteins, are a rich source of vitamins, minerals, and antioxidants that help reduce inflammation and support liver function. Additionally, because soups contain a high water content, they aid in hydration, which is important for the processes involved in liver detoxification. Finally, the warmth and comfort of soups can soothe the digestive system and improve nutrient absorption.

Contrarily, salads are usually made up of raw, fresh ingredients that retain all of their nutritional value. Leafy greens, which are frequently the foundation of salads, are rich in chlorophyll, which helps to promote the production of bile, which is necessary for the breakdown of fats and the removal of toxins from the body. Additionally, the fiber in salads aids in digestion and prevents the accumulation of toxins in the liver by encouraging regular bowel movements.

A well-rounded approach to maintaining and improving liver health can be created by incorporating a variety of these ingredients into your diet through soups and salads. Certain ingredients that are particularly beneficial for liver health can be added to both soups and salads. These include citrus fruits that provide vitamin C for immune support and cruciferous vegetables like broccoli and Brussels sprouts that enhance liver detoxification enzymes.

COMFORTING AND FILLING SOUP RECIPES

Rich, filling soups are a great way to incorporate a variety of foods that are good for the liver, such as protein and fiber from lentils and vitamins and antioxidants from various vegetables. To make this soup, sauté onions, garlic, and celery in olive oil until soft. Add diced carrots, tomatoes, and bell peppers. Stir in lentils, vegetable broth, and your preferred herbs, such as bay leaves and thyme. Simmer until the lentils are tender, and you have a rich, filling soup.

Lean protein and cleansing greens are also found in chicken and kale soup. To make the soup, first, sauté chopped onions, garlic, and carrots in a big pot. Next, add diced chicken breast and cook until browned. Next, add low-sodium chicken broth and bring to a boil. Finally, add chopped kale, potatoes, and a small pinch of turmeric for anti-inflammatory effects. Simmer the soup until the chicken is cooked through and the vegetables are soft, then taste and adjust the seasoning with salt and pepper.

A more unusual option is to make a miso soup with tofu and seaweed. Miso is fermented soybean paste, which has probiotics that are good for the liver and gut. To make the soup, first bring water to a boil, then add a few pieces of kombu (edible kelp) for flavor. After a few minutes, remove the kombu and dissolve the miso paste in the hot water. Next, add cubed tofu, sliced mushrooms, and chopped green onions.

Simmer for a short while, then stir in some wakame seaweed, which is high in vitamins and minerals.

SIMPLE AND INVIGORATING SALAD RECIPES

Salads are a great way to get essential nutrients without the heavy weight of cooked meals. One classic example is a spinach and citrus salad, which combines the vitamin C from citrus fruits with the liver-cleansing properties of leafy greens; start with a base of fresh spinach leaves, then add grapefruit and orange segments; toss in some thinly sliced red onions and pomegranate seeds for extra antioxidant action; and dress with a light vinaigrette made with lemon juice and olive oil.

Cucumber and avocado salad is another hydrating and low-calorie option that is great for liver health. To make it, thinly slice the cucumbers and avocados, then add cherry tomatoes, fresh dill, and a squeeze of lime juice. Gently mix and season with a pinch of salt and pepper.

This salad is not only low-calorie and nutrient-dense, but it also contains healthy fats from the avocado that are vital for liver function and nutrient absorption.

This salad is packed with protein, fiber, and a variety of vitamins and minerals that support overall liver health. If you're looking for something more substantial, try a quinoa and vegetable medley. Cook the quinoa according to the package instructions and let it cool. Then, in a large bowl, combine the quinoa with diced bell peppers, cherry tomatoes, cucumbers, and chopped parsley. Add a handful of crumbled feta cheese for a touch of creaminess. Dress with a mixture of olive oil, lemon juice, and a hint of garlic.

HOW TO PREPARE WELL-BALANCED SALADS

Incorporating a range of food groups and textures is key to making satisfying, well-balanced salads. Begin with a base of leafy greens, like spinach, arugula, or mixed salad greens, which offer vital vitamins and minerals. Add a colorful assortment of vegetables, like bell peppers, carrots, and beets, to this base to boost antioxidants and fiber content. Adding a variety of colors ensures that the salad has a wide range of nutrients.

After that, add a source of lean protein to make the salad more substantial and well-balanced. Lean protein aids in muscle repair and prolongs feelings of fullness. You can also add a source of healthy fat, like avocado, nuts, seeds, or a drizzle of olive oil. Healthy fats are essential for the absorption of fat-soluble vitamins (A, D, E, and K) and also add flavor and texture to the salad.

Finally, add complex carbs like quinoa, farro, or sweet potatoes to your salad. These foods offer long-lasting energy and fiber that helps with digestion and keeps you full. Use herbs and spices like basil, cilantro, or black pepper to add flavor without going overboard with calories. Steer clear of high-calorie toppings like croutons or too much cheese and instead choose nutrient-dense options that add to the salad's overall nutritional profile.

Simple vinaigrette made with olive oil, balsamic vinegar, Dijon mustard, and a dash of honey can be made at home; just whisk the ingredients together and season with salt and pepper.

This dressing is versatile and goes well with most salads, adding a tangy and slightly sweet flavor without overpowering the other ingredients. Store-bought dressings are often loaded with added sugars and preservatives.

Try this yogurt-based dressing for a creamy alternative: whisk together plain Greek yogurt, lemon juice, minced garlic, and fresh herbs such as parsley or dill. This dressing has less fat than traditional creamy dressings and adds tangy flavor and probiotics that are good for gut health. Another great option is a tahini dressing, which is made by combining tahini (sesame seed paste) with lemon juice, water, and a little garlic. It tastes nutty and savory and is rich in healthy fats.

Additions to salads can improve their flavor and nutritional value. Nuts and seeds, like cranberries, walnuts, and sunflower seeds, add a satisfying crunch and are rich in protein and healthy fats. Dried fruits, like raisins or butternut squash, can offer some sweetness and extra fiber. Roasted vegetables, like butternut squash or beets, can make a substantial and flavorful topping. These additions not only improve the flavor and texture of your salad but also provide essential nutrients that support liver health.

SNACKING ON DESSERTS WHILE TAKING CARE OF YOUR LIVER

Desserts can still be a part of a balanced diet for those who manage their liver health. The key is to choose desserts that will satisfy your sweet tooth without overloading your liver with nutrients. Desserts made with whole grains, fruits, and healthy fats can provide nutrients without taxing your liver.

Yogurt parfaits with fresh berries or baked apples with cinnamon can be delicious options that support liver function. You can enjoy desserts while prioritizing liver health by emphasizing moderation and nutrient density.

RECIPES FOR NATURALLY SWEETENED DESSERTS

Selecting naturally sweetened dessert recipes can be advantageous for both taste and health. Sweeteners such as honey, maple syrup, or dates can provide sweetness without the refined sugars that can tax the liver.

Desserts like mashed banana-sweetened chia seed pudding or nut-date oatmeal cookies are satisfying substitutes for traditional desserts that not only ease the load on your liver but also add extra fiber and nutrients. Try these recipes to enjoy dessert guilt-free while supporting the health of your liver with healthy ingredients.

LOW-SUGAR AND LOW-FAT SELECTIONS

A balanced approach to dessert consumption that benefits your liver is ensured by choosing low-fat and low-sugar dessert options. For example, fruit sorbets made with little added sugar or angel food cake topped with fresh fruit can satisfy cravings without adding excessive fats or sugars.

These choices help to maintain stable blood sugar levels and lower the risk of fat accumulation in the liver. Desserts that are light and nutritious allow you to enjoy treats while supporting liver function and overall health.

USING FRUITS IN DESSERT RECIPES

Fruits have a wealth of vitamins, minerals, and antioxidants that support liver function and overall well-being. By creatively utilizing fruits in desserts, you can enjoy natural sweetness without added sugars that can strain the liver. These options provide a delicious way to indulge in desserts while prioritizing liver-friendly ingredients. Fruit salads with a drizzle of yogurt or grilled peaches topped with a sprinkle of cinnamon can be refreshing and satisfying dessert ideas.

SOME ADVICE ON PORTION CONTROL

Use smaller dishes or bowls to visually control portions and prevent overindulging. Additionally, concentrate on nutrient-dense desserts that satisfy cravings without needing large quantities. Dark chocolate-dipped strawberries or a small serving of Greek yogurt with a drizzle of honey can be satisfying treats that support liver health.

LIVER-FRIENDLY COCKTAIL SELECTIONS

Drinking water is one of the best drinks for liver health because it helps flush toxins from the body and supports liver function. You can add a slice of lemon or cucumber to enhance the detoxifying effect and add a refreshing twist. Liver-friendly drink options are crucial for supporting liver health and aiding in its detoxification processes. These beverages are designed to be gentle on the liver, helping to reduce inflammation and promote overall wellness.

Herbal teas such as dandelion root tea or milk thistle tea are also beneficial. Dandelion root tea supports liver detoxification by stimulating bile production, while milk thistle tea contains silymarin, a potent antioxidant that helps protect liver cells from toxins. Green tea is another great option because it is rich in catechins, which are antioxidants that help protect liver cells from damage and promote healthy liver function.

Finally, coconut water is a hydrating option that provides electrolytes and minerals, making it a good choice for liver support. Its natural sweetness makes it a pleasant alternative to sugary drinks, which should be avoided.

Ginger tea is a great option for those looking to add more flavors. Ginger has anti-inflammatory properties and can aid digestion, which indirectly supports liver health. It's easy to prepare by steeping fresh ginger slices in hot water.

RECIPES FOR HOMEMADE JUICES AND SMOOTHIES

A simple juice recipe consists of carrots, beets, and apples. Beets contain betaine, a compound that aids in the removal of toxins from liver cells. Apples add sweetness and fiber, aiding in detoxification. Homemade juices and smoothies can be great additions to a diet that is friendly to the liver, as they provide essential nutrients without the added sugars and preservatives.

Blend spinach, kale, cucumber, and banana to create a nutrient-rich smoothie. Leafy greens like spinach and kale are rich in antioxidants and chlorophyll, which support liver detoxification processes.

Cucumber adds flavor and hydration, and the banana offers natural sweetness and potassium, which helps the body maintain fluid balance. A tablespoon of ground flaxseed or chia seeds can increase omega-3 fatty acids, which are anti-inflammatory and good for liver health.

Mango offers vitamins and antioxidants; pineapple contains bromelain, an enzyme that aids in digestion and reduces inflammation; and coconut water adds electrolytes and a tropical flavor without added sugars. These homemade drinks are not only delicious, but they also support liver health by providing essential nutrients and hydration, which is crucial for detoxification. Mango, pineapple, and coconut water make for a tropical twist on smoothies.

In addition to its calming effects on the digestive system, which indirectly support liver function by promoting proper digestion and reducing bloating, peppermint tea is a popular choice after meals due to its refreshing taste.

Another beneficial herbal tea is chamomile, which has anti-inflammatory properties and can help relax the body and mind. This gentle tea is ideal for promoting relaxation while supporting overall liver health. Herbal teas and infusions offer a soothing and therapeutic way to support liver health and detoxification.

Due to its strong anti-inflammatory and antioxidant qualities, turmeric tea is becoming more and more popular. Curcumin, the compound that makes up turmeric, protects liver cells from harm and supports the liver's detoxification pathways. Another effective option is ginger tea, which is made from fresh ginger root.

Ginger promotes liver function, aids in digestion, and reduces inflammation. It can be steeped in hot water or brewed fresh.

Consider less common options like dandelion root tea or milk thistle tea. Dandelion root tea stimulates bile production, which aids in digestion and supports liver detoxification processes. Both herbal teas can be enjoyed throughout the day as part of a liver-friendly diet to promote overall wellness. Milk thistle contains silymarin, a powerful antioxidant that protects liver cells from toxins and promotes regeneration.

DRINKS THAT REHYDRATE AND DETOXIFY

Water with a splash of lemon or cucumber is a simple yet effective way to stay hydrated while supporting liver detoxification. Lemon helps alkalize the body and aids in digestion, while cucumber adds a refreshing flavor and helps flush out toxins. Hydration is key to liver health, and incorporating hydrating and detoxifying drinks into your daily routine can support optimal liver function.

A squeeze of lime can enhance the flavor of coconut water and add extra vitamin C, which supports immune function and detoxification. Coconut water is naturally low in calories and sugars, making it a healthier alternative to sugary drinks that can burden the liver. It contains electrolytes like potassium and magnesium, which support cellular function and hydration levels.

Try a fruit and herb-infused detox water for a more decadent treat that still supports liver health. Just cut up some strawberries, mint leaves, and cucumber slices, then add them to a pitcher of water and let it infuse overnight in the refrigerator. This infused water tastes great and is a great way to stay hydrated and support overall wellness. It also contains antioxidants and vitamins that support liver detoxification.

AVOIDING SUGAR-SUGARY DRINKS AND ALCOHOL

Since alcohol is metabolized by the liver and excessive consumption over time can cause fatty liver disease, liver inflammation, and even cirrhosis, it is imperative to limit or avoid alcohol completely to protect liver cells and support overall liver function. Reducing alcohol intake and sugar-filled drinks is also important for preventing liver disease.

Drinks high in added sugars, such as soda, energy drinks, and sweetened juices, can also be detrimental to the liver. They can cause insulin resistance, weight gain, and fatty liver disease. A better option for promoting liver health is water, herbal teas, or homemade juices and smoothies. It's important to read labels and make choices that have little to no added sugar.

Prioritizing hydration and selecting drinks that nourish your body without taxing your liver is a proactive step toward maintaining optimal liver health. Avoiding alcohol and sugary drinks in favor of hydrating, nutrient-rich beverages can support liver health and promote overall wellness. Small changes to your beverage choices can have a significant impact on liver function and lower the risk of liver disease over time.

CHAPTER SIX

PARTICULAR DIETARY REQUIREMENTS

HANDLING ADDITIONAL MEDICAL CONDITIONS

Taking a holistic approach to diet is important when managing liver disease in conjunction with other health conditions. Conditions such as diabetes or hypertension can have a significant impact on liver health and necessitate careful dietary choices.

For example, people with diabetes should control their blood sugar levels by avoiding refined sugars and carbohydrates. Lean proteins, whole grains, and healthy fats can help stabilize blood sugar levels and support liver function. People with hypertension should limit their intake of sodium to lower their risk of fluid retention and further liver damage. Choosing fresh fruits, vegetables, and herbs as flavor enhancers rather than salt can help manage both conditions concurrently.

RECIPES FREE OF GLUTEN AND GOOD FOR LIVER

For those with liver disease who also have gluten intolerance or celiac disease, a gluten-free diet is essential. Wheat, barley, and rye should be avoided while naturally gluten-free grains such as quinoa, rice, and corn are included. These recipes typically include fresh vegetables, lean proteins, and healthy fats to support liver function and overall health. For example, a gluten-free stir-fry made with quinoa provides essential amino acids and fiber without causing gluten-related inflammation. By using gluten-free flour like almond or coconut flour in baking, people can enjoy treats like gluten-free liver-friendly muffins or bread without violating their dietary restrictions.

VEGAN AND DAIRY-FREE SELECTIONS

Dairy-free and vegan liver-friendly options include adding legumes, tofu, tempeh, and nuts as protein sources. Calcium-rich substitutes like fortified plant-based milk and leafy greens like kale and broccoli support bone health without relying on dairy products. Vegan liver-friendly recipes often emphasize fresh produce, whole grains, and healthy fats to provide essential nutrients and promote liver detoxification. For instance, a dairy-free smoothie made with almond milk, spinach, berries, and chia seeds provide antioxidants, fiber, and omega-3 fatty acids beneficial for liver health.

RECIPES LOW IN SODIUM

To manage fluid retention and lower the risk of complications like ascites or edema, people with liver disease must limit their intake of sodium. Low-sodium liver-friendly recipes emphasize the use of herbs, spices, and citrus juices to enhance flavors without the need for salt. For example, a low-sodium vegetable stir-fry seasoned with garlic, ginger, and lemon juice offers a savory alternative to salt-heavy dishes. Adding fresh herbs, such as parsley, cilantro, or basil to salads and soups helps further elevate flavors while providing antioxidants and essential nutrients. Adding potassium-rich foods like bananas, sweet potatoes, and leafy greens to salads and soups helps balance sodium levels and support overall liver function.

CUSTOMIZING RECIPES TO MEET SPECIFIC NEEDS

Customization is key to making sure meals are both enjoyable and supportive of liver health. For instance, replacing wheat pasta in a traditional pasta dish with gluten-free alternatives or zucchini noodles accommodates gluten intolerance while providing essential vitamins and minerals. Similarly, substituting plant-based proteins for animal proteins in recipes like burgers or tacos caters to vegan or vegetarian preferences without compromising protein intake. Adding or omitting ingredients based on individual tolerances and nutritional goals ensures that liver-friendly meals are per person's specifications.

CHAPTER SEVEN

DINING OUT AND SOCIAL OCCURRENCES

DINING OUT AND SOCIAL OCCURRENCES

ADVICE ON EATING OUT WHILE HAVING LIVER DISEASE

Choosing from a menu can be intimidating for people with liver disease, but it can be done with some planning. Look for restaurants that offer healthy options or can accommodate special dietary needs. A lot of places now offer nutritional information online, which makes decision-making easier.

When at the restaurant, choose dishes that are grilled, baked, or steamed rather than fried to cut down on fat intake. Ask for sauces and dressings to be served on the side to control portions.

To facilitate better digestion and avoid discomfort, take your time when eating and eat slowly. Pay attention to portion sizes because large meals can put a strain on the liver. If you have any questions about the ingredients or the preparation process, don't be afraid to ask your server for clarification.

Finally, enjoy your meal by focusing more on the company and conversation than the food.

SELECTING HEALTHFUL MENU ITEMS AT RESTAURANTS

Selecting dishes with heavy sauces or creamy dressings—which often contain excess fat and calories—avoids dishes that incorporate fresh vegetables or salads with vinaigrette dressing on the side. Whole grains, like brown rice or quinoa, are preferred over refined carbohydrates, like white bread or pasta. Managing liver disease at restaurants requires making healthy choices. To start, scan the menu for lean protein options, like grilled chicken or fish, which are easier on the liver.

Drink water, herbal tea, or sugar-free fresh fruit juices to stay hydrated and cut down on extra calories. Stay away from alcohol entirely as it can worsen liver damage. If you're having a buffet or ordering several courses, control portion sizes by starting with a small salad or soup and not overindulging.

Finally, pay attention to your body's signals of hunger and fullness to ensure a balanced meal and promote liver health.

GETTING AROUND AT PARTIES AND SOCIAL EVENTS

Planning and practicing mindfulness is key to navigating social events and parties with liver disease. Eat a small, wholesome meal or snack before the event to help you curb your appetite and prevent overindulging in less healthful options. At the event, look over the food options and select dishes that fit your dietary needs, like salads, grilled proteins, or vegetable-based dishes; politely decline offerings that are fried, heavily sauced, or high in sugar and sodium.

Plan and be mindful to ensure that you enjoy the social aspect of the event while making conscious choices that support your well-being. Participate in conversations and activities to take your mind off food and lessen the temptation to overindulge. If alcohol is served, choose mocktails without alcohol or sparkling water with lemon to participate in toasts and socialize without endangering the health of your liver.

MAKING LIVER-FRIENDLY RECIPES FOR PARTIES

Making liver-friendly food for parties can be fulfilling and supportive of your diet. To begin, look for recipes that highlight lean proteins, like turkey, chicken, or fish, as these are less taxing on the liver. Add lots of fresh fruits and vegetables to your dishes to supply vital nutrients and fiber. Use cooking techniques like baking, grilling, or steaming to reduce added fats and oils while maintaining flavor.

Try enhancing the flavor of your food with herbs, spices, and citrus juices instead of depending too much on heavy sauces or seasoning. Make sure to serve a range of appetizers and side dishes to suit the tastes and dietary needs of your guests. Let them know in advance about any dietary requirements or preferences you may have to meet their needs and protect your health.

Managing your dietary needs in social situations requires effective communication. Before you go to any meetings or events, let the host or organizer know about your dietary needs and preferences. Offer to bring one or two dishes that meet your needs so that you can enjoy yourself worry-free. When you talk to people about your dietary needs, be succinct and straightforward about what you can and cannot eat.

At mealtimes, ask nicely about ingredients or cooking techniques to make sure that food is prepared in a way that promotes liver health. Thank them for any accommodations they have made for you and provide an alternative if needed. Keep in mind that speaking up for your health is not only essential but also encourages others to think about dietary inclusivity. When you are open and courteous with others, you can enjoy social events without sacrificing your health.

CHAPTER EIGHT

SUSTAINING NUTRITIONAL ROUTINES OVER TIME

CREATING LONG-TERM ROUTINES

Developing long-lasting eating habits is essential to effectively managing liver disease. Begin by determining the major dietary adjustments that are required, such as cutting back on sodium and saturated fats while increasing foods high in fiber. Include a range of fruits, vegetables, whole grains, and lean proteins in your daily meals. Introduce these changes gradually to give your body time to adjust and facilitate the shift. Use portion control to control your intake of calories and maintain a healthy weight, which is critical for the health of your liver.

Plan your meals and make them at home with fresh ingredients if you want to maintain these habits over time. Steer clear of processed foods and sugary drinks because they can aggravate the symptoms of liver disease.

Drink lots of water to stay hydrated. Get regular exercise, like swimming or walking, to support your general health and boost your energy levels. Finally, ask for help from family, friends, or a dietitian to help you stay motivated and accountable when implementing these new habits.

MONITORING DEVELOPMENT AND REMAINING INSPIRED

The key to effectively managing liver disease is tracking your dietary progress. Use apps or websites to track your nutrient intake, ensuring you meet dietary recommendations for liver health. Regularly assess your weight, energy levels, and overall well-being to gauge the impact of your dietary changes. Keep a food journal to keep track of what you eat and how it makes you feel. This can help identify foods that trigger symptoms or discomfort.

Setting realistic goals and acknowledging small victories along the way will help you stay motivated. Reward yourself with non-food items or enjoyable activities.

Participate in online communities or support groups devoted to liver health to exchange stories and get advice from others going through similar struggles. Learn about liver disease and how to manage your diet to appreciate the significance of your efforts. Keep in mind that while progress may vary, maintaining consistent healthy habits is essential for long-term success.

HANDLING OBSTACLES

Any health condition, including liver disease, has setbacks. If you experience a setback in your diet, such as overindulging in unhealthy foods or skipping workouts, don't be too hard on yourself. Instead, consider what caused the setback and use it as a chance to sharpen your resolve. Reassess your goals and, if necessary, adjust your strategies to get back on track.

Seek assistance from medical professionals, dietitians, or counselors who can offer direction and support during trying times. Remind yourself that obstacles are only temporary and that you can regain momentum toward better health with perseverance. Concentrate on the improvements you've made and use them as inspiration to keep moving forward toward successfully managing liver disease.

ONGOING INSTRUCTION AND ASSISTANCE

Maintaining long-term health requires ongoing education about liver disease and diet management. Get informed about the most recent findings, available treatments, and dietary guidelines from credible sources, such as medical journals, trustworthy websites, or healthcare providers. Participate in liver health-focused webinars, seminars, or workshops to broaden your knowledge and network with professionals in the field.

You can feel empowered to make decisions about your health and well-being by staying informed and supported. Seek out ongoing support from healthcare professionals, dietitians, or support groups to address any questions or concerns you may have. Talk to others about your experiences to gain encouragement and insights. Join online forums or social media groups dedicated to liver disease to stay connected with a community of people on similar journeys.

SOURCES FOR ADDITIONAL READING AND ASSISTANCE

Locating trustworthy sources for additional reading and assistance can improve your comprehension and handling of liver disease. Seek out books, articles, or websites written by medical experts with expertise in liver health.

These sources frequently offer comprehensive details on dietary recommendations, treatment choices, and lifestyle advice for liver disease sufferers.

Look into online discussion boards, support groups, or liver-related social media groups to get in touch with people who have gone through similar things. These platforms provide a place to ask questions, exchange ideas, and get advice from others who have been through similar things. You can also attend in-person or online support groups run by patient advocacy groups or healthcare providers to get more information and direction.

For the most recent information on managing liver disease, visit credible websites like those run by government health agencies, universities, or medical centers. These websites frequently have articles, fact sheets, and patient guides that can add to your knowledge and give you the confidence to make health-related decisions. However, always seek advice from medical professionals or dietitians before making major dietary or treatment plan modifications based solely on information you find online.

CHAPTER NINE

IF I HAVE ADDITIONAL MEDICAL CONCERNS, CAN I STILL ADHERE TO THIS DIET?

A liver disease diet should be evaluated for any other medical conditions you may have. Its main goal is to lessen the stress on the liver by eliminating foods that are hard on it, such as processed foods high in sodium, alcohol, and fats. However, if you have other medical conditions, such as diabetes or hypertension, you may need to make some adjustments. For example, if you have diabetes, you may need to watch how much sodium you consume, even when following the liver disease diet's guidelines.

For the same reason, if you have hypertension, you may need to monitor your sodium intake even when following the liver disease diet's recommendations. Speaking with a dietitian or your primary care physician can help.

HOW SHOULD I RESPOND IN THE EVENT OF A FLARE-UP?

A flare-up of liver disease symptoms can be difficult, but there are things you can do to manage it within the parameters of your diet. First, you should review the fundamentals of the liver disease diet, emphasizing the consumption of easily digested foods that are gentle on the liver. This includes foods high in fiber, like fruits, vegetables, and whole grains, which can help with digestion and promote liver function. Secondly, you should stay hydrated to support liver health and overall well-being.

Finally, you should avoid triggers like alcohol, fatty foods, and processed foods during a flare-up to prevent further stress on the liver. Finally, you should closely monitor your symptoms and seek advice from healthcare providers to ensure that your liver is taken care of.

HOW CAN I MAINTAIN MY MOTIVATION TO FOLLOW THE DIET?

Planning meals ahead of time and keeping a variety of liver-friendly recipes on hand can make it easier to stick to the diet consistently. Regular physical activity, which is beneficial for liver health, can further motivate you to maintain a healthy lifestyle. Joining support groups or asking for encouragement from friends and family can provide additional motivation and accountability. Remember that adhering to a liver disease diet requires commitment and motivation, especially when faced with temptations or challenges. One effective strategy is to focus on the positive outcomes of following the diet, such as improved liver function, increased energy levels, and overall well-being.

ARE THERE ANY SUPPLEMENTS THAT I MIGHT TAKE TO AID MY LIVER?

A balanced diet for liver disease may benefit from the use of supplements, but it's important to use them sparingly and under the supervision of a professional.

Milk thistle, for instance, is well-known for its liver-protective qualities; it contains active ingredients like silymarin that may promote liver cell regeneration. Vitamin E, on the other hand, has antioxidant properties that may help reduce oxidative stress in the liver.

Nevertheless, before taking any supplements, it's important to speak with a healthcare provider because they may interact with medications or exacerbate certain medical conditions. Healthcare providers can recommend the proper dosage and oversee their effects on liver health, making sure they support rather than contradict the

IF I EAT ANYTHING THAT ISN'T GOOD FOR MY LIVER, WHAT SHOULD I DO?

Eventually, you will inevitably come across foods that are incompatible with a diet for liver disease. In this case, you should not panic but rather take proactive measures to minimize any potential damage to your liver.

First and foremost, after consuming a non-liver-friendly food, make sure you stay well hydrated by drinking lots of water. This will help flush toxins from your system and support liver function. You should also think about including foods that cleanse the liver, like leafy greens, cruciferous vegetables, and antioxidant-rich fruits like berries. You should also consider including liver-cleansing foods in your subsequent meals, such as leafy greens, cruciferous vegetables, and berries. Light physical activity can also help with digestion and promote overall liver health. Finally, avoiding alcohol and high-fat foods in your subsequent meals can help your liver recover.